MW01144641

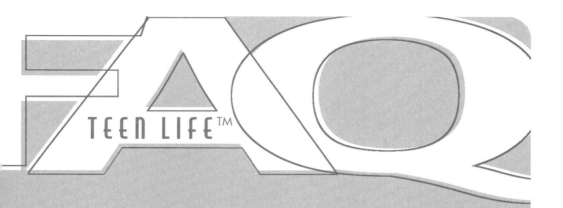

TEEN LIFE™

FREQUENTLY ASKED QUESTIONS ABOUT

AIDS and HIV

Richard
Robinson

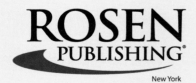

ROSEN
PUBLISHING®

New York

Published in 2009 by The Rosen Publishing Group, Inc.
29 East 21st Street, New York, NY 10010

Library of Congress Cataloging-in-Publication Data

Robinson, Richard, 1956–
Frequently asked questions about AIDS and HIV / Richard
Robinson.—1st ed.
    p. cm.—(FAQ: Teen life)
Includes bibliographical references.
ISBN-13: 978-1-4042-1808-6 (library binding)
1. AIDS (Disease)—Miscellanea—Juvenile literature. 2. HIV
infections—Miscellanea—Juvenile literature. I. Title.
RC606.65.R63 2008
616.97'92—dc22

                                                    2008001116

Manufactured in the United States of America

Contents

1 What Are HIV and AIDS? 4

2 Where Did AIDS Originate? 9

3 How Is the AIDS Virus Contracted? 14

4 What Can You Do to Stay Safe? 23

5 How Do You Deal with a Positive Diagnosis? 36

6 How Can I Live a Fulfilling Life with AIDS/HIV? 46

Glossary 56
For More Information 58
For Further Reading 60
Index 62

WHAT ARE HIV AND AIDS?

The Joint United Nations Program on HIV/AIDS estimates that there were 40.3 million people around the world living with HIV at the end of 2005. Of these, approximately 1.2 million lived in the United States. Sadly, more people become infected with the virus each year, and others who were already infected die from AIDS. According to the Centers for Disease Control and Prevention (CDC), roughly 13 percent of the people diagnosed with HIV or AIDS in 2004 and 5 percent of those who died of AIDS were between the ages of thirteen and twenty-four.

Since it was first recognized in 1981, AIDS has killed 25 million people. "It is the worst and deadliest disease that humankind has ever experienced," according to Mark Stirling, UNAIDS director of East and Southern Africa. What's worse, there is no cure for—or vaccine against—AIDS.

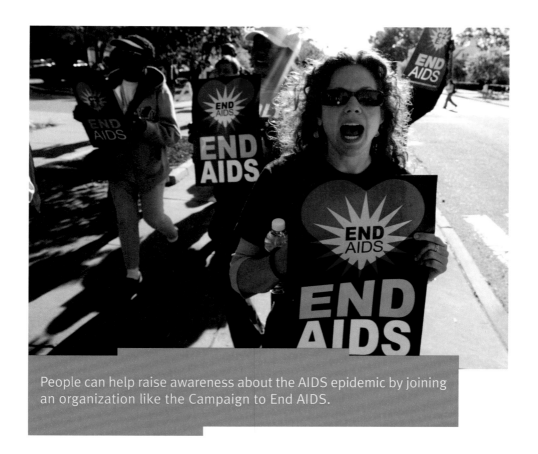

People can help raise awareness about the AIDS epidemic by joining an organization like the Campaign to End AIDS.

Although these statistics are frightening, you are not powerless against AIDS. It is true that HIV/AIDS is a growing danger for everyone, but it is a danger we can understand and avoid. As medical researchers scramble to find a cure, it is important to remember that AIDS is preventable. Taking the proper precautions to prevent infection is the first step in fighting this disease that affects so many people.

There is still a lot of ignorance and misinformation about AIDS. Replace these with useful knowledge. Scientists and researchers are working hard to make this disease extinct. You can play your part by learning how to protect yourself and the people you care about from AIDS.

AIDS Defined

HIV is a virus that attacks the body's immune system, making it unable to fight infection. The National Institutes of Health (NIH) defines AIDS as the most serious stage of HIV infection that results from the destruction of the infected person's immune system. The CDC further explains the disease by defining each word in its name as follows:

- "Acquired" means the disease is not hereditary, but develops after contact with a disease-causing agent (in this case, HIV).
- "Immunodeficiency" means the disease is characterized by a weakening of the immune system.
- "Syndrome" refers to a group of symptoms that characterize a disease. In the case of AIDS, this can include the development of certain infections and/or cancers, as well as a decrease in the number of certain cells in a person's immune system.

A Positive Outlook

It can be discouraging to realize that even modern medicine cannot eliminate a disease from the world, but the news isn't all bad. Thanks to therapies that have been developed over the last

See **BEYOND FEAR**

Where: _____
Dates: _____ Time: _____

You Can't Get AIDS—

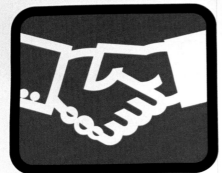

By Shaking Hands

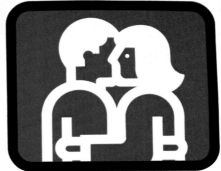

Or By Hugging

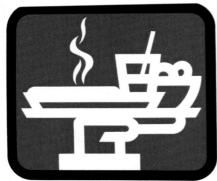

In Restaurants

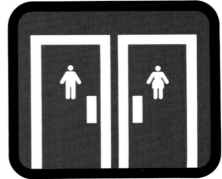

Or In Restrooms

**AIDS doesn't spread through casual contact.
Don't let fear get in the way of facts.
Take the time to learn about AIDS.**

American
Red Cross

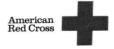

Funding provided by
American
Council of
Life
Insurance

HEALTH
INSURANCE

National Red Cross
merly AIDS-11)

Myths about how AIDS can be contracted create a lot of fear.
The American Red Cross is working to keep people informed of the
truth about AIDS.

decade, many people who are currently infected with HIV live longer, healthier lives than those from the first group of people who contracted the virus. Moreover, there are many things that can help a person with HIV or AIDS to live well, from taking certain medicines to eating well, exercising, and getting rest. The support of family and friends is also a big help.

HIV is not as easy to catch as a cold or the flu, or hepatitis, tuberculosis, or polio. All of those diseases can be passed from one person to another by shaking hands, sharing food, or breathing on each other. HIV is a much more delicate virus. It is not airborne. It does not live outside of the human body. When it gets cold or dries up, HIV dies.

WHERE DID AIDS ORIGINATE?

During the late 1970s and early 1980s, doctors became aware that an increasing number of people were suffering from several rare illnesses. One of these illnesses was a respiratory disease, Pneumocystis carinii pneumonia (PCP), which was usually a problem only for cancer patients undergoing chemotherapy. Another was a rare skin cancer, Kaposi's sarcoma, which, until then, mostly affected Mediterranean or Jewish men over fifty years old who would usually live for years after diagnosis. However, the men becoming ill with these diseases were much younger and had previously been healthy. The diseases progressed so rapidly within their bodies that it appeared as if their immune systems were no longer working to resist them. Consequently, the men became weak and died. The number of cases recognized by doctors in cities across the United States grew from a few dozen in 1980 to several thousand within five years.

The Early Victims

At first, very little was known about what was happening. Who was becoming ill? Was this a disease caused by a germ or the result of drug abuse? Would it spread among people at work or school or in cities?

Many of the first few people diagnosed with this condition were homosexual men. As a result, the condition was referred to as gay-related immunodeficiency, or GRID. However, it also showed up in intravenous drug users—male and female—who weren't homosexuals.

Another group of people affected by the disease were hemophiliacs. These people (almost all male) have a rare condition from birth that makes it hard for their blood to clot. They need to have regular injections of a clotting factor derived from blood donations. None of the infected hemophiliacs abused intravenous drugs, and few were homosexuals. Soon, the wives of some infected hemophiliacs became ill, and that further alarmed the medical community.

It became clear that the illness was contagious. It was being passed from the sick men to their sexual partners, both male and female. Another clue lay in the fact that intravenous drug abusers sometimes share needles, which can bring a drop of blood from one person to another. It became obvious that the illness must be caused by something that could be carried in

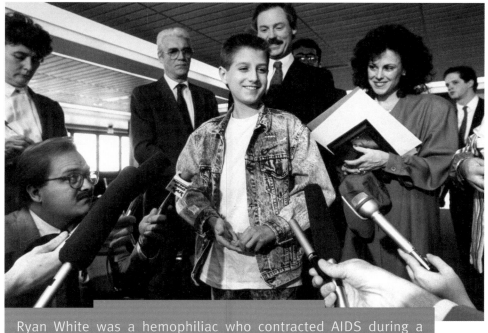

Ryan White was a hemophiliac who contracted AIDS during a blood transfusion. Before his death in 1990, White worked to raise awareness about the AIDS epidemic.

blood. Doctors checked among patients who had received blood transfusions or organ donations and found a few other people who were affected by this new disease.

Solving the Mystery

It took research in hospitals and laboratories all around the world to figure out what was happening: a previously unknown and rare disease had spread from person to person. The virus made a person's immune system stop working so that he or she

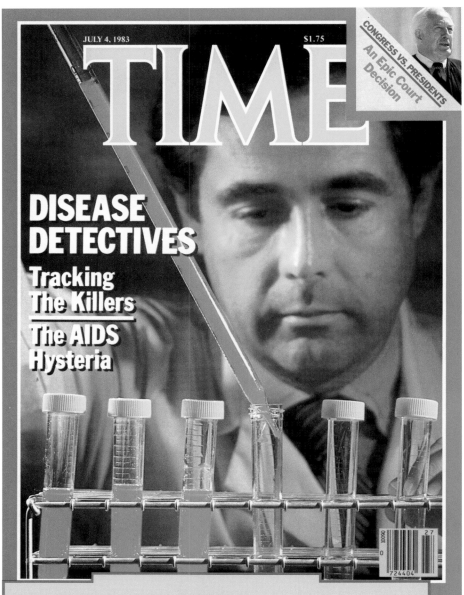

Time magazine helped to bring attention to the AIDS crisis with this issue, which came out on July 4, 1983. The cover photo was taken at the Centers for Disease Control and Prevention (CDC).

would become ill from multiple causes and die. It was as if a person had acquired the very rare illness of being born with little or no immune system. In 1982, this disease was named acquired immune deficiency syndrome, or acquired immunodeficiency syndrome (AIDS).

In 1983, the Institut Pasteur in France recognized that a virus was the cause of AIDS. This virus was named human immuno-deficiency virus (HIV). Researchers now understood how the virus moved from one person to another by the exchange of semen, blood, or vaginal secretions during sexual contact, or by coming into contact with the blood of an infected person—most likely through needle sharing and blood transfusions. Researchers learned how HIV weakens the body's immune system by attacking specific white blood cells called T-helper cells, or CD4 cells.

Another breakthrough was the achievement in 1985 of a test for HIV antibodies in the blood. If a person has HIV, his or her immune system makes antibodies to try to kill the virus. Developing this test was crucial because a person with HIV might not look or feel ill for many months or years, and may therefore unwittingly pass the disease to others.

three

HOW IS THE AIDS VIRUS CONTRACTED?

HIV is spread primarily by sexual contact that involves an exchange of bodily fluids. According to the CDC, 80 percent of all HIV/AIDS cases diagnosed in the United States in 2004 were the result of sexual contact. The gender of the people touching does not matter. The virus can be transmitted from a man to a woman, from a woman to a man, from a man to a man, or from a woman to a woman. Nevertheless, males account for 73 percent of American adults and adolescents living with HIV/AIDS.

If a male who has HIV does not wear a condom, the virus in his semen and pre-seminal fluid could infect his partner. A female who has HIV could infect her partner with the virus from her vaginal fluids. Any tiny cut or sore inside a vagina, anus, mouth, or on a penis would make it easy for the virus to pass into a person's body. A tiny sore like this is usually too small to see or feel.

HIV is also transmitted by coming into contact with an infected person's blood, most likely by sharing needles during injection drug use. Close to 20 percent of all Americans living with HIV/AIDS were infected this way. A pregnant woman who is HIV positive can pass the virus to her unborn child. While the incidence of children being born with HIV is only fractional in the United States, the rates are significantly higher in other parts of the world where anti-HIV therapies are not readily available.

Situations That Will NOT Lead to an HIV Infection

- Touching a doorknob that has been touched by a person who is HIV positive
- Insect bites
- Being friends with, or working with, a person who is HIV positive
- Touching a toilet seat that has been used by a person who is HIV positive
- Donating blood
- Swimming in a pool with a person who is HIV positive
- Sharing food or drink with an HIV-positive person, or even drinking from the same straw

The Genetics of HIV

Like other viruses, HIV cannot grow or reproduce on its own. A virus must infect the cells of a living organism—a person, animal, or plant—in order to make new copies of itself.

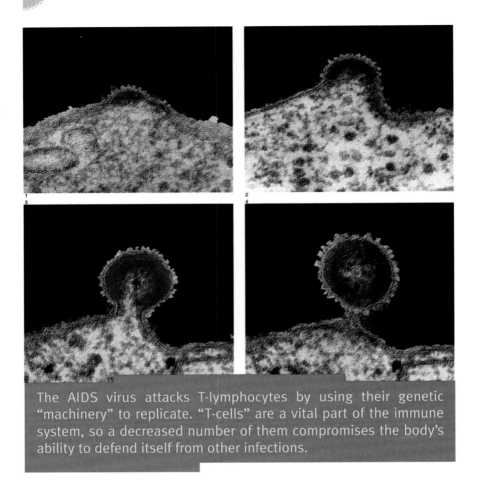

The AIDS virus attacks T-lymphocytes by using their genetic "machinery" to replicate. "T-cells" are a vital part of the immune system, so a decreased number of them compromises the body's ability to defend itself from other infections.

HIV is one of a special class of virus called retroviruses. A retrovirus uses a reverse version of some standard enzymes in our cells. Almost all organisms, including most viruses, store their genetic material on long molecules of DNA (deoxyribonucleic acid). But the genes of retroviruses are made of RNA (ribonucleic acid). RNA has a very similar structure to DNA.

HIV has just nine genes. That's not many compared to the more than five hundred genes in some bacteria, or around twenty thousand to twenty-five thousand genes in a human. These genes can mutate, making tiny changes in the virus.

Inside Human Cells

When a virus gets inside a living cell, it uses the cell's own copying process to make copies of itself. When this process is hijacked by a lethal virus such as HIV, the result is a lot of copies of the virus and a dead cell.

HIV uses chemicals called enzymes to get into a cell, hide itself there, and get copies of itself made. Once inside a human cell, HIV uses an enzyme, reverse transcriptase, to convert its own viral RNA into DNA. In the cell's nucleus, this DNA is spliced into the human DNA by another HIV enzyme, called integrate. That integrated HIV DNA may remain dormant within a cell for a long time.

But when the cell becomes activated to make new proteins for many uses, it treats the HIV genes much like human genes. First, the cell uses human enzymes to convert the genes into messenger RNA, and then the RNA is transported outside the nucleus to be a blueprint for producing new proteins and enzymes. Some of these RNA strands are complete copies of HIV, which are released from the cell in particles ready to infect other cells.

What Are the Symptoms?

A person who is HIV positive can live for years without developing any symptoms. But there are some common warning signs of HIV infection. If you experience any of these symptoms, do not be alarmed. It does not mean that you have HIV. Many other illnesses have similar symptoms. The symptoms of HIV infection are not unique. They just show that a person's immune system is being stressed. It's up to a doctor to diagnose the illness that is causing the symptoms.

Swollen lymph nodes are early warning signs of HIV infection. Lymph nodes are part of the immune system. They are small, bean-shaped organs that are also called glands. You can sometimes feel them in your neck, armpits, and groin. Other nodes are deep inside the body. Lymph nodes store immune cells, which can trap and destroy bacteria and viruses that enter the body. A lymph node swells as the immune cells inside attack foreign invaders.

Other possible warning signs of HIV infection include a flu-like illness (usually experienced within weeks after exposure to HIV), frequent fevers, excessive sweating, unexplained fatigue, rapid weight loss, pneumonia, breathing difficulties, or diarrhea that lasts longer than a week. A person with HIV could develop white spots or sores in the mouth and throat, or blotches on or under the skin that are red, pink, purple, or brown.

Stages of HIV and AIDS

The CDC recognizes several steps in the progression from HIV infection to AIDS. They are:

- **Infection:** The earliest stage is right after you are infected. HIV can infect cells and copy itself before your immune system has started to respond. You may have felt flu-like symptoms during this time.
- **Response:** The next stage is when your body responds to the virus. Even if you don't feel any different, your body is

trying to fight the virus by making antibodies against it. This is called seroconversion, when you go from being HIV negative to HIV positive.

→ **No symptoms:** You may enter a stage in which you have no symptoms. This is called asymptomatic infection. You still have HIV, and it may be causing damage that you can't feel.

→ **Symptoms:** Symptomatic HIV infection is when you develop symptoms such as certain infections, including Pneumocystis carinii pneumonia.

→ **AIDS:** AIDS is diagnosed when you have a variety of symptoms, infections, and specific test results. There is no single test to diagnose AIDS.

Life Expectancy

Some people progress quickly from infection with HIV to showing symptoms after only a few months. They may die within two years, usually from an illness that takes advantage of the immune system failure. This is more common in places where there is little medical care, but it can happen anywhere.

In the United States, where medical care is available and people usually enjoy good health and nutrition, the news is somewhat better. Some people stay asymptomatic for many months or years. In 2004, the CDC found that only 39 percent of Americans diagnosed as HIV positive in 2003 received an AIDS diagnosis in fewer than twelve months. For a while, once a person was diagnosed with AIDS, he or she usually lived for less than two years. However, the CDC also found that among Americans diagnosed with AIDS after 2000, 90 percent survived

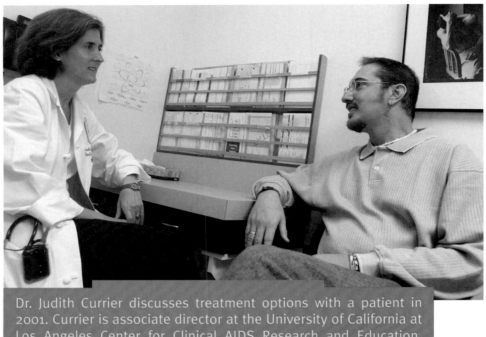

Dr. Judith Currier discusses treatment options with a patient in 2001. Currier is associate director at the University of California at Los Angeles Center for Clinical AIDS Research and Education, where experimental medical trials are conducted.

for more than a year, 86 percent survived for more than two years, and 83 percent survived for more than three years. The main reason for these amazing survival rates is the development of retroviral drugs over the last decade.

Myths and Facts

 AIDS is only a problem for gay people. Fact ➻ HIV/AIDS is something for everyone to know about, whether they are homosexual or heterosexual. Even people who never have sex may someday need a blood transfusion, and they will be glad to receive blood that has been tested for HIV antibodies.

 AIDS is only a problem in crowded cities. Fact ➻ AIDS is a problem wherever people are. People can be exposed to HIV one time and after that can bring the virus inside their bodies wherever they travel.

 If I abuse drugs, I can't get AIDS unless I share a needle with another user. Fact ➻ Drug abusers can become infected with HIV by sharing needles or doing other high-risk activities while they are under the influence of the drugs. Drug abusers can have plenty of diseases and health problems, even when they don't share needles. They are also at risk for dangerous behavior and violent crimes.

If young people learn anything about sex, they are more likely to have sex and get AIDS. Fact ●→ Sexual health education helps young people understand their bodies and how to stay healthy.

Maybe a sick person with AIDS could get cured by having sex with a virgin. Fact ●→ Nothing cures AIDS. If a person with any disease has sex with a virgin, that does not cure the disease. It may even give the disease to the virgin.

Once people get AIDS, they are going to die soon. Fact ●→ Some people who have HIV can live for years with good medical care and nutrition. They can even enjoy moderately good health and most normal activities. Some have lived fifteen years or more without progressing to a diagnosis of AIDS.

chapter four

WHAT CAN YOU DO TO STAY SAFE?

AIDS is not a disease that gets better and goes away. It cannot be cured by medicine or beliefs or clean living. The only defense against AIDS and HIV is prevention, and the only way to prevent the spread of AIDS is to avoid the behaviors that transmit HIV from person to person. Chief among these are unprotected sex and intravenous drug use.

Whatever type of birth control you choose, it should offer dual protection. First, it should protect against pregnancy. But second—and just as important—it should protect against potentially deadly sexually transmitted diseases, such as AIDS (which is caused by HIV), as well as gonorrhea, chlamydia, and others. Effective contraception must serve these two critical purposes.

Avoiding High-Risk Behavior

It can be difficult to say no to sex or drug use, but avoiding these two behaviors is how we can protect ourselves from disease. Your decisions should be respected by your friends, boyfriend or girlfriend, and family. You have the right to protect your life—and the lives of people you care about—by saying no.

If you decide to have sex, be smart about it. You cannot tell whether your partner has HIV. In many cases, he or she might not know either. Unprotected sex is risky. Using latex condoms means that HIV has fewer chances of being transmitted during sexual contact.

Post-exposure prophylaxis (PEP) is recommended for people thought to have been exposed to HIV. PEP reduces your chances of contracting HIV. While health-care workers are the most common recipients of PEP, people who have had sex with an infected person, either voluntarily or by rape, should also undergo PEP.

The most common PEP program is one drug, or a combination of several, taken for four to six weeks. Doctors recommend starting PEP as soon as you think you have been exposed, but you can start the program up to seventy-two hours after exposure. Studies show that the sooner you start PEP, the more effective it is at reducing your risk of contracting HIV.

If you think you may have been exposed to HIV, whether through sexual contact or a dirty needle, call your doctor immediately.

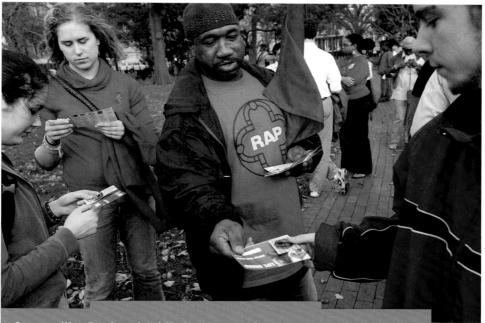

Groups like Regional Addiction Prevention, Inc., create awareness by handing out free condoms and information about HIV and AIDS on World AIDS Day.

Unprotected Sex

HIV is most commonly spread by bodily fluids—blood, semen, and vaginal secretions—during sexual contact. It can be passed sexually from male to female, from male to male, from female to male, and rarely from female to female. The virus is most likely to be transmitted by contacting bodily fluids with an open sore or a break in the skin.

Sexual contact includes anything involving a penis, vagina, anus, or mouth. Most methods of safe sex involve using a condom or dental dam as a barrier to prevent contact with bodily fluids. Unprotected sexual contact means that no barrier is used. Even the first time a person has sex, it's important to have protected sex. Also, the more sexual partners a person has, the more likely he or she will have sex with someone who is HIV positive. If both partners are HIV positive, they should still have protected sex to avoid being infected with different versions of HIV.

Sharing Needles

HIV can be spread when people who abuse intravenous drugs share needles. Roughly 20 percent of all HIV infections are caused this way, but that's only half of the picture. According to the CDC, "Injection drug use contributes to the epidemic's spread far beyond the circle of those who inject. People who have sex with an injection drug user (IDU) also are at risk for an infection through the sexual transmission of HIV. Children born to mothers who contracted HIV through sharing needles or having sex with an IDU may become infected as well." The CDC estimates that injection drug use has directly or indirectly contributed to about 36 percent of AIDS cases in the United States. Other diseases, like hepatitis C, can be transmitted this way, too. Moreover, injecting illegal drugs is generally unsafe and hazardous to your health. Among other things, you risk a deadly overdose.

People can avoid this risk of AIDS completely by not using injection drugs. For those who cannot or will not stop using drugs, it is important that they not share needles and syringes or use them more than once. There are many programs that help drug abusers quit using drugs and/or provide clean needles.

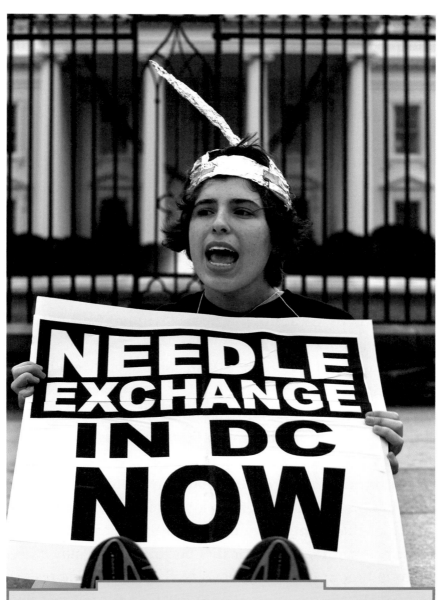

A protester demonstrates for needle exchange programs to be put in place. Drug users can contract HIV by using the same needle as someone who is HIV positive.

The CDC notes that the abuse of non-injection drugs also contributes to the spread of AIDS. In one study of two thousand young adults in three inner-city neighborhoods, the agency found that smokers of crack cocaine were three times more likely to be infected with HIV than non-smokers. People often make bad decisions, including engaging in risky sexual behaviors, when they are high.

Having Safer Sex

Abstinence, or not having sexual intercourse, is the only sure way to avoid getting HIV by sexual contact. However, if you're going to have sex, then it is important to practice safe sex. Sexual touching does not have to be high-risk behavior. Kissing, touching with hands, and rubbing bodies will not transmit HIV from one person to another.

Intercourse is much less likely to transmit the virus if a barrier is used. A barrier is usually a latex condom or dental dam. Avoid condoms that are made from animal membranes because germs can get through them. A lubricating cream or jelly should be used, one that kills HIV and is spermicidal (kills sperm). This will make the barrier less likely to break. However, if the barrier breaks, the lubricant will be there to kill sperm or the virus. The lubricant should be water-based. It is unsafe to use Vaseline, baby oil, and cooking oil as lubricants because these may cause the condom to break.

AVERT, a UK-based international HIV and AIDS charity, advises against the use of condoms and lubricants that contain a spermicide called nonoxynol-9, which was once thought to help prevent the spread of HIV, but has since been proved ineffective. Nonoxynol-9 kills sperm and is the active ingredient in most over-the-counter spermicides. But nonoxynol-9 does NOT protect you from contracting the HIV virus (which causes AIDS) or other sexually transmitted diseases like gonorrhea or chlamydia. And while nonoxynol-9 can be used alone in cream or gel form, it is also used as a spermicide within condoms. But there is also no evidence that condoms lubricated with nonoxynol-9 are any more effective in preventing pregnancy or infection than condoms lubricated with silicone, according to the World Health Organization (WHO). Last, frequent use of vaginal contraceptives with nonoxynol-9 can also cause vaginal irritation and lesions (small cuts) in the vaginal wall, which can actually increase the likelihood of HIV infection. For all these reasons, many members of the medical community advise against the use of nonoxynol-9 as a means of birth control.

A male should put a latex condom on his penis before touching a partner's vagina, mouth, anus, or penis. Anything that enters a person's vagina, mouth, or anus should be covered with a condom. Partners should not share sex toys with each other or anyone else.

Traditionally, condoms have been made from latex. But you may have seen newer polyurethane condoms, too. Some people claim that polyurethane condoms are more sensitive than latex ones because they are thinner in texture. But studies show that polyurethane condoms are not as effective in protecting against pregnancy and sexually transmitted diseases. Polyurethane condoms are more likely to slip off the penis during withdrawal and also to break. The bottom line is, unless you are among the

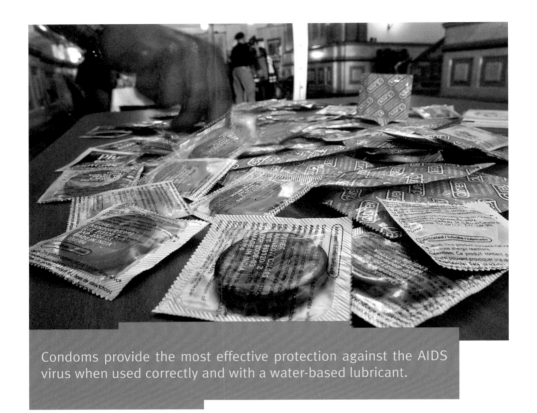

Condoms provide the most effective protection against the AIDS virus when used correctly and with a water-based lubricant.

small number of people allergic to latex, latex condoms are a far safer option.

A female should use lubricant if her male partner is using a condom. A female could also use a lubricant and a female condom to line her vagina if her male partner is not using a condom.

If a female is using a diaphragm, cervical cap, or sponge for birth control, even with lubricant this is not enough protection for safe sex. These methods of birth control block sperm from entering a woman's uterus, but they would not block HIV from entering tiny sores inside her vagina.

A person who is allowing a penis, finger, or anything else to enter her or his anus should use lubricant, as the anus is easily damaged. Any tiny sores would allow HIV into the body.

A dental dam is a sheet of latex that can be used between a female's vagina and a person's mouth, or between an anus and a mouth. If you can't find dental dams at a store, make one by unrolling a condom and cutting it open along one side to make a flat sheet of latex. Although the lubricant may not taste good, it is safe to get in the mouth during sex.

Fidelity Is Low-Risk Behavior

For some people, the preferred option for low-risk behavior is fidelity, meaning both partners choose to have sex only with each other. One of the best reasons for not having sex outside of marriage or other committed relationships is being sure that each partner will not bring an HIV infection—or other disease—to the other. As for being sure about your partner, this behavior choice relies on trust and keeping promises.

HIV Testing

It takes a doctor's diagnosis to recognize HIV or AIDS. This is done with a simple blood test. A person who has been infected with HIV will test positive for the antibody. Such a person is said to be HIV positive.

Everyone should know his or her HIV status—especially those who engage in, or have engaged in, high-risk behavior. There's no need to worry if you might be HIV positive—get

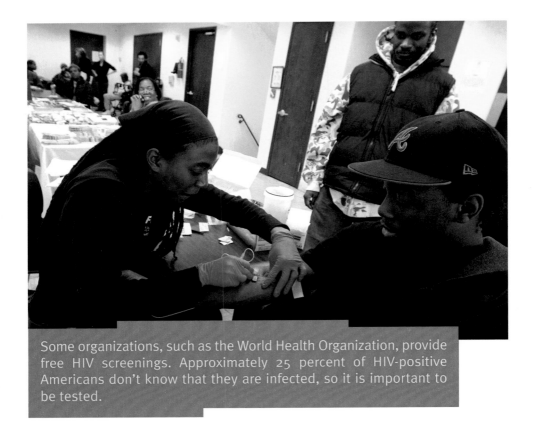

Some organizations, such as the World Health Organization, provide free HIV screenings. Approximately 25 percent of HIV-positive Americans don't know that they are infected, so it is important to be tested.

tested and you'll know for sure. The test for HIV antibodies is very reliable and available.

According to the CDC, approximately 25 percent of Americans who are HIV positive do not know they are infected. Research also shows that most people who know they are infected take steps to reduce their risk of infecting others. Given these two realities, it makes sense that increasing the number of people who know their HIV status can help to reduce HIV transmission. In addition, more HIV-positive individuals would get the treatment they need. Accordingly, the CDC recommends that HIV testing become part of routine medical examinations.

The Tests

It's easy to get tested for HIV. Generally, a small amount of blood is drawn from your arm using a sterilized syringe. This blood test takes only a few minutes, and you'll feel just a small poke with the needle.

The blood is sent to a laboratory to be tested. The results will be made known to you after one to three weeks. There are different places you can go to get tested, and the test can be done anonymously or confidentially.

Places for Testing

You can choose one of many places to go for an HIV test. Hospitals, clinics, private doctors' offices, family planning or sexually transmitted disease clinics, health departments, and mobile sites offer HIV testing. Some of these places charge for a test, while others offer it for free. After you decide where you want to be tested, choose either an anonymous test or a confidential test.

Anonymous and Confidential HIV Testing

If you take an anonymous HIV test, you do not have to give your name. A unique code will be used to identify you instead. The only person who will know your actual test results is you. This type of test is available in most states.

You can also use an at-home test, or collection kit, to be anonymous. This test can be ordered over the phone or the Internet, and it will be shipped to you. You have to take a sample of your own blood, as explained in the kit, and send it to a

At-home AIDS tests can be ordered from a legitimate source over the phone or Internet in order to keep your results anonymous.

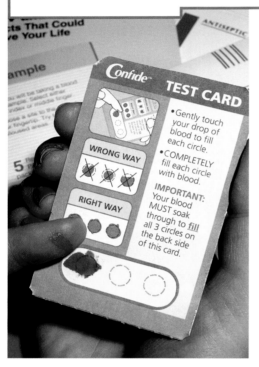

laboratory. The results will be sent to you in a few weeks. They are not given to anyone else, and most are considered quite accurate.

Before you purchase a kit over the phone or Internet, research the type of kit and its brand online. And be careful which brand you buy because scams are out there. Make sure that the kit is legitimate and approved by the FDA (Food and Drug Administration).

Notwithstanding the convenience of the home tests, most experts advise people to have their HIV tests done in a medical setting, where counseling is a part of the process. Most people dread the thought of being HIV positive and are therefore extremely anxious about taking the test. Counseling helps to allay these anxieties, particularly if the result comes back positive.

Confidential HIV testing is also called names testing. Unlike anonymous HIV testing, you are required to give your name, and the result is released only to the medical personnel who administered the test and, in some states, the state health department. You can choose to have the results added to your medical record. All states make this type of HIV test available.

Responsibility

Being tested for HIV is a way to take responsibility for your own life and actions. It's a smart choice that helps you take control of your health care. It can be scary to wait for test results and the potential consequences, but knowing the truth can help you make good choices.

HOW DO YOU DEAL WITH A POSITIVE DIAGNOSIS?

Learning that you are HIV positive may be the most devastating news that you can receive. However, realize that, unlike when it was first discovered, HIV is not a death sentence. Many people, including basketball great Magic Johnson, go on to live long, productive lives after they discover their HIV-positive status. You can, too.

A positive HIV test doesn't mean you have AIDS, but HIV can progress to AIDS if it remains untreated. Therefore, some of the first things you should do after learning your status is to find out more about the disease, find support, and see an HIV doctor. Chances are that if you did your HIV test in a medical setting, the doctor, nurse, or counselor there would have given you some information about how to go about doing these things.

Testing positive for HIV can be a terrifying and isolating experience. It is important to be able to confide in a loved one.

Telling a Loved One

Many people recall feeling terribly alone when they first tested positive for HIV. Although this is a normal reaction, it is important to recognize that there is an incredible network of support organizations that offers aid, information, and comfort to HIV-positive individuals. No matter how willing these

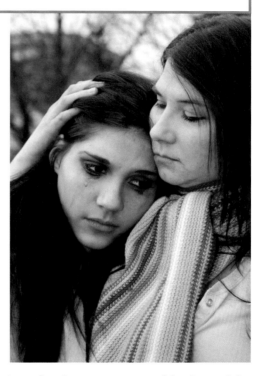

groups are to help, they recognize the importance of being able to share your diagnosis with someone you trust, especially if that person is a loved one. "Connecting with others . . . while you're adjusting to the news is one of the 'first steps' we recommend," says Regan Hofmann, editor-in-chief of *POZ* magazine.

Ideally, teenagers who test positive for HIV without their parents' knowledge should inform their parents right away. It is generally unwise to keep such a critical diagnosis from the very people who are most responsible for your well-being. Although teenagers may be tested for HIV without parental consent, they need such consent to obtain treatment.

Enlist the help of someone else, like a counselor from the clinic where you did the test, to break the news to your parents if you feel you cannot face them alone. You're likely to find that your parents will rally to your support no matter how shocked they are by the news. If, however, your parents are not supportive, choose someone else whom you think will be able to handle the news and keep your secret. Although it is difficult to tell how people will respond, you should have an idea of who will be there for you.

Regardless of the support you get from your family, consider joining a support group for people who are recently diagnosed with HIV. (There are support groups for parents of HIV-positive people, too.) Such groups can be instrumental for easing your anxieties, providing you with reliable information, and steering you in the right direction for the various services, including medical treatment, that you may need.

Finding a Doctor

See an HIV doctor as soon as possible after receiving an HIV-positive diagnosis. The initial test only determines your HIV status. You'll need to undergo further tests to find out how the virus is affecting your body and how soon you'll need treatment. HIV care is ongoing. Unless a cure is found, you'll likely see your doctor every three or four months for the rest of your life. Therefore, it is important that you find the right doctor for you.

Finding a doctor is not difficult. Your current primary care doctor may be an HIV specialist, or he or she may be able to refer you to one. You can also seek the advice of other HIV-positive people, a support group, AIDS services organizations, or the clinic or medical center where you did the test.

Your First Doctor Visit

Your first visit to the HIV specialist is crucial. You'll be establishing a relationship with someone with whom you'll be working to make informed decisions about your treatment for a very long time, perhaps for the rest of your life. It's likely that you'll be anxious. The doctor will anticipate this and try to reassure you that, despite your diagnosis, you can lead a healthy and productive life. This is a good time for you to ask questions, so you may want to jot down whatever questions you may have and take them with you to the appointment.

In addition to asking you questions about your medical history, the doctor will do a physical examination and order a number of blood tests. These tests will help your doctor to determine how the virus is affecting your body and whether you'll need to start treatment soon. The two standard tests include a CD4 count and a viral load test. The CD4 count reports the number of CD4 cells, or T cells, in a sample of your blood. The higher the count, the better the result, since CD4 cells are the white blood cells that fight infection, but are targeted by the HIV virus. The viral load test measures the amount of HIV in a sample of your blood. It shows how well your immune system is controlling the virus. The lower the load, the better the result. Together, the CD4

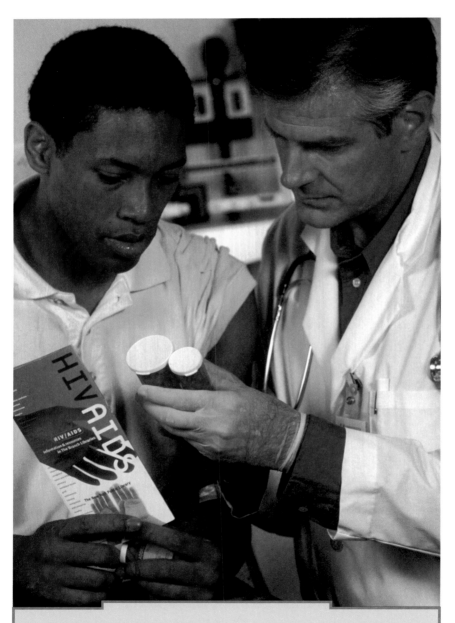

It is extremely important to find an HIV specialist whom you can trust with your care after your initial diagnosis.

count and the viral load count provide a baseline (or initial) measurement for future tests.

Your doctor is likely to order drug resistance tests, which determine whether someone's HIV has developed resistance to any anti-HIV medication. You may wonder how your virus could be resistant to anti-HIV medications before you've taken them. Drug resistance is transmitted along with the virus. In other words, you will inherit whatever drug resistance the person who infected you with HIV has. Your doctor may do other tests, including:

- A complete blood count (CBC), which checks all the different blood cells
- A blood chemistry profile, which shows how well your liver and kidney are working, and measures the lipids (fats) and sugar (glucose) in your blood
- Tests for other sexually transmitted diseases (STDs)
- Tests for other infections such as hepatitis, tuberculosis, or toxoplasmosis
- Pregnancy test and a Pap smear (for females)

Beginning Treatment

Depending on the results of these blood tests, you and your doctor will determine when you should start treatment and what medication to take. Not every one who tests positive for HIV begins treatment right away. However, left untreated, HIV progresses into AIDS in an average of ten years. This rate of progression is a general estimate. HIV affects everyone differently. For a few people, referred to as the elite, HIV never progresses to AIDS. The National Institutes of Health (NIH) recommends beginning treatment if:

→ You are experiencing severe symptoms of HIV, or have been diagnosed with AIDS.

→ Your viral load is 100,000 copies/mL or more.

→ Your CD4 count is 200 cells/mm3 or less.

→ You and your doctor may decide to begin taking medication before these criteria are met.

Medicines That Help

Anti-HIV medications are known as antiretroviral medications. These medications are used to control the reproduction of the virus, thereby slowing the progression of HIV-related disease. To date, the FDA has approved twenty-two antiretrovirals, which fall into four categories based on how they work against HIV.

1. Nonnucleoside reverse transcriptase inhibitors (NNRTIs) interrupt the first step HIV takes to copy itself by binding to and disabling reverse transcriptase, a protein necessary to the copying process.

2. According to the FDA, nucleoside reverse transcriptase inhibitors (NRTIs) "are faulty versions of building blocks that HIV needs to make more copies of itself. When HIV uses an NRTI instead of a normal building block,

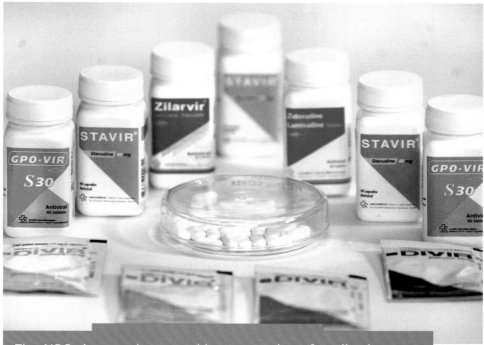

The AIDS virus can be treated by any number of medications or a combination of medicines. Antiretroviral medications control the reproduction of the virus and slow the progression of the disease.

reproduction of the virus is stalled." Like the NNRTIs, NRTIs also interrupt the first step HIV takes to copy itself.

3. Protease inhibitors (PIs) interrupt the last stage HIV takes to copy itself by disabling protease, a protein necessary for the copying process.

4. Fusion inhibitors work by blocking HIV from entering into cells. The FDA, to date, has approved only one drug in this class: Fuzeon (enfuvirtide).

Follow-Up Visits to Your Doctor

Especially after you begin taking antiretroviral medications, you will be required to visit your doctor every three or four months so that he or she can monitor how well your treatment is working. During these visits, your doctor will order a CD4 count and a viral load test to measure against the baseline measurements that were established during your first visit. He or she will monitor your general health as well.

You should use these scheduled visits to further develop your relationship with your doctor. When he or she asks you how things are going, be prepared to give a full account of your health over the last few months. Consider making a list of the questions and issues you want to raise with your doctor. It may help you to keep a diary, noting things like missed doses or major changes in your life that affect your stress levels.

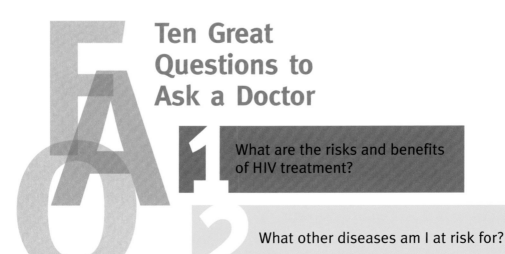

Ten Great Questions to Ask a Doctor

1 What are the risks and benefits of HIV treatment?

2 What other diseases am I at risk for?

3 How can I avoid transmitting HIV to others?

4 How can I achieve and maintain a healthier lifestyle?

5 What should I do if I miss a dose of my HIV medication?

6 What should I do if I have problems sticking to my treatment regimen?

7 Can I infect someone else if my viral load is undetectable?

8 What are the likely side effects of the medications I take? Which side effects are serious?

9 Will the side effects go away by themselves? Are there any side effects that should prompt me to stop taking my medication?

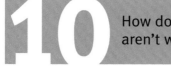

10 How do I know if the drugs aren't working anymore?

HOW CAN I LIVE A FULFILLING LIFE WITH AIDS/HIV?

Finding out that you're HIV positive will definitely change your life. Especially after you begin treatment, HIV will factor into your everyday schedule in many ways. But your HIV status need not dominate your life. The sooner you get used to your new routine, the better you can enjoy the rest of your life. There are things you can do to maintain or improve your quality of life. Perhaps the most important things are making sure that you stay healthy, developing a good support system, pursuing your dreams, and making time for fun.

Diet and Exercise

Eating well and exercising are good for everyone. They are even more essential for HIV-positive individuals, whose immune systems are constantly under assault by the virus. Becoming familiar with the U.S. Department of

The first step toward remaining healthy is to achieve a balanced diet that includes lots of fruits and vegetables.

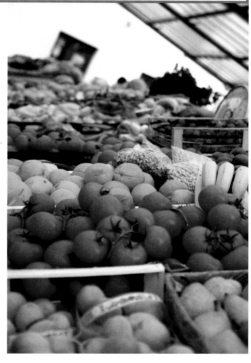

Agriculture's Food Guide Pyramid is a good place to start on your way to eating healthy. The pyramid shows that a balanced diet includes all the major food groups, but emphasizes certain foods (fruits, vegetables, grains, and dairy) over others (meat and oils). The pyramid also recommends at least thirty minutes of moderate-to-vigorous physical activity every day. Moderate exercise includes walking briskly, dancing, and bicycling. Vigorous exercise includes running, swimming, and basketball.

Avoiding Risky Behaviors

Good general health includes avoiding risky behavior. Being HIV positive doesn't give you a free pass to continue or start sharing needles during drug use or having unprotected sex. On the contrary, having HIV is a strong reason not to engage in these behaviors. In addition to exposing others to infection, you run the risk of superinfection, which is becoming infected with another strain of HIV. Superinfection increases the likelihood of your developing resistance to anti-HIV medication, which will reduce the treatment options available to you.

Moreover, drug abuse, whether or not it involves needles, impairs a person's judgment. A person who abuses drugs may end up doing other dangerous things as well. There is the risk of overdose and immediate death. A person who abuses drugs is at greater risk of being beaten or raped, of catching diseases, or of being injured. These are avoidable risks.

A person's immune system may be weakened by drug abuse. This can make it easier to become ill with many kinds of diseases. Drug abuse can interfere with the medicines prescribed by a doctor. Be honest with your doctor about any substance use, whether it's a lot or a little, and whether it's alcohol, illegal drugs, misused prescription drugs, or marijuana. Even cigarettes and tobacco, though legal, are addictive and have profound health effects. If you are abusing intravenous drugs or any substance, consider seeking help.

How to Protect Others

If you are HIV positive, you have a responsibility not to infect other people with the virus. Be honest about your HIV status. People who care about you deserve to know this. It's hard to risk rejection, but being honest is being responsible.

➡ Tell your sexual partner that you are HIV positive.

➡ Do not have unprotected sex, even if you previously had unprotected sex with this person.

➡ Tell people with whom you have had sex that you are HIV positive.

➡ If you hope to have a new sexual partner, tell this person you are HIV positive before becoming intimate.

➡ Do not share your razor or toothbrush with anyone.

➡ If you become pregnant, or if you are thinking about having a child, talk to your doctor right away.

➡ If you abuse drugs, do not share needles. More important, get help for your addiction.

Getting and Giving Support

There are support groups for people living with AIDS and HIV. Support groups can bring you great comfort as you meet people who share similar experiences. Just knowing that other people are facing the same challenges can help you feel less isolated or lonely.

The people in a support group are people like yourself, whose lives are affected by HIV and AIDS. They can help you understand treatment methods and ways to adjust your lifestyle. One of them will have some training as a facilitator and be able to help you find resources or the answers to questions.

It can make you feel isolated and alone if you are HIV positive and have not told your family. If you're scared of what they will say, or you are not ready to share, that's understandable. A support group can help you prepare yourself for how you will tell your friends and family.

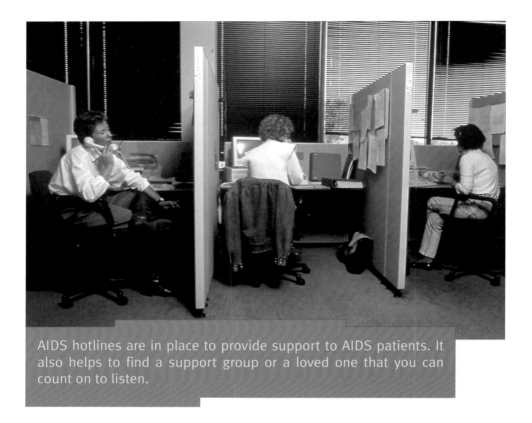

AIDS hotlines are in place to provide support to AIDS patients. It also helps to find a support group or a loved one that you can count on to listen.

You can be affected by AIDS even if you are not the person infected with HIV. Finding out that someone you care about is HIV positive is upsetting. Support groups help friends and family as well, not just the person who is HIV positive.

Physical Care

A person who is HIV positive but asymptomatic may not need much physical help. For someone who is at an early symptomatic stage, there may be times when he or she needs assistance for daily living. On occasion, the care of a trained nurse may be needed, but friends or family can learn how to care for the majority of a person's physical needs.

By the time a person is diagnosed with AIDS, there will be good days and bad days, but the person may likely need physical care much of the time. Family members and friends can take turns helping. Or, perhaps one helper will concentrate on one aspect such as running errands and doing laundry, while another will look after nursing care.

The changes in what a person is physically able to do can be upsetting for everyone. It can also be an opportunity to recognize that we all live in real bodies, bodies that change with time and health and chance. There will certainly be emotional reactions, too.

Emotional Effects

It is emotionally exhausting when anyone in a household is ill. When illnesses go on for months or years, the entire household must make adjustments and plan ways to renew each person's emotional strength. Take time to restore your own energy, and make sure everyone in your household does the same. This is one way you can help each other. You can also give each other space to feel better.

Support groups can be a great help. A support group may suggest ideas that worked in other households. Members may offer validation that your emotional reactions are realistic, not whining or selfish or unreasonable. Sometimes, part of the solution is just knowing that other people are going through similar experiences.

What Difference Can I Make?

You are only one person. But each day you can do something positive to make that day better. Even small improvements can be special.

You may be able to work with a circle of family and friends to accomplish things that make your lives better. You may be part of a larger project or political movement that influences the lives of many. Anything that changes the world happens because of the actions of individual people.

You have the ability to be nice to the people who live in your home. A kind word, helping someone with homework or housework, telling a funny story, or listening to someone else's news are all things that show you care. They can be done by a person who usually needs the most help from others.

Disclosing Your HIV Status

Being HIV positive isn't something that will be obvious to everyone. Even having AIDS is not as visible as losing an arm or using a wheelchair. It is a health difference that doesn't show, and it's up to you to decide what difference it makes in the ways you behave with the people you meet. You don't need to tell anyone about your HIV status, though telling those with whom you've had sex or you're planning to have sex is the responsible thing to do. You don't have to tell your school. If you choose to disclose your HIV status, bear in mind that you risk rejection.

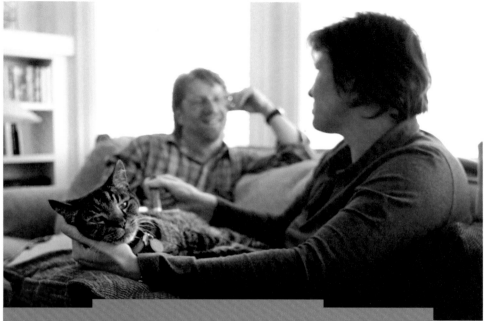

There are a lot of things volunteers can do to help out. This PAWS (Pets Are Wonderful Support) volunteer helps an AIDS patient care for his cat. His compromised immune system prevents him from being able to go near the litter box because of germs.

It's not your job to educate everybody you see about AIDS and HIV, but it doesn't hurt to think ahead. What would you say if someone asked you a question? How could you help a stranger who had an accident? When is it best to be anonymous?

Some days you will make different decisions about what to say and what actions to take. But you can always use your knowledge about HIV and AIDS to help you be confident that you are making good decisions for your health and community.

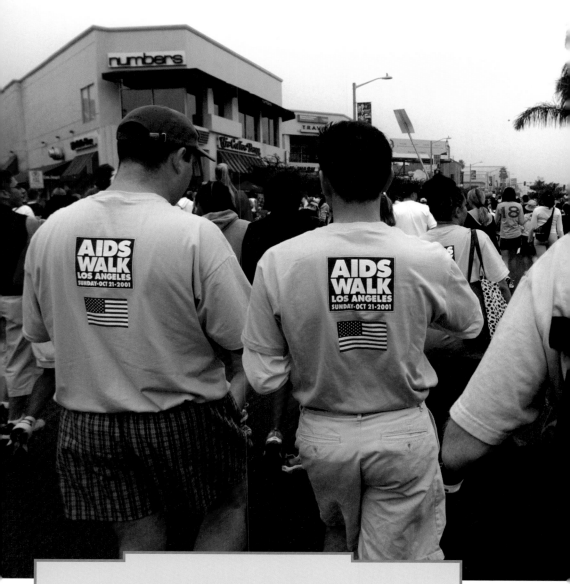

The AIDS Walk gives individuals a chance to raise money for AIDS research by finding sponsors to fund the walk.

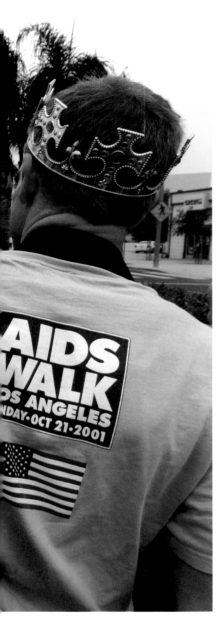

Being an Example

Some things about AIDS and HIV are private. There are also times when it is proper to speak in public about AIDS, go to a meeting, or march in a parade. A loop of red ribbon pinned on a shirt or jacket is a visible reminder that you care.

There are activities you can do in your community to show support for people with HIV or AIDS. There are educational programs. Some communities have events to raise money for a local clinic or hospice. Other programs send money overseas to support people with HIV or their orphaned children. Your small acts in support of HIV/AIDS causes can make a big difference in the lives of others who are living with the disease.

Glossary

abstinence Avoidance of sexual contact.

acquired Not hereditary, but develops after contact with a disease-causing agent.

antibody A protective protein produced by the immune system in response to the presence of a foreign substance.

antigen A foreign substance, when introduced into the body, can stimulate an immune response.

confidential Kept secret to protect a person's privacy.

enzymes Proteins that bring about specific biochemical reactions in the body.

epidemic Affecting a large number of people within a population, community, or region at the same time.

hemophilia Genetic blood defect that causes a delayed clotting of the blood that can lead to difficulty in stopping blood loss, even in the case of minor injury.

immune system System that protects the body from foreign substances, cells, and tissues.

immunodeficiency Characterized by a weakening of the immune system.

lymphocyte A white blood cell that determines how the immune system will respond to the presence of an antigen.

retrovirus Virus that reproduces in the body by replicating within the body's DNA.

superinfection Infection by more than one strain of the
HIV virus.

syndrome Group of symptoms that characterize a disease. In
the case of AIDS, this can include the development of certain
infections and/or cancers, as well as a decrease in the
number of certain cells in a person's immune system.

Information

AIDS.gov

U.S. Department of Health and Human Services

200 Independence Avenue SW

Washington, DC 20201

Web site: http://www.aids.gov
  The government service that provides reliable resources
  on AIDS and HIV.

AIDS Walk New York

Old Chelsea Station

P.O. Box 10

New York, NY 10113

Web site: http://www.aidswalk.net
  An organization that works to raise funds for AIDS research.

Global Network of People Living with HIV/AIDS

P.O. Box 11726

1001 GS Amsterdam

The Netherlands

Web site: http://www.gnpplus.net
  An organization that fights for the rights of people living
  with HIV and AIDS.

The Names Project Foundation

AIDS Memorial Quilt

637 Hoke Street NW

Atlanta, GA 30318

(404) 688-5500

Web site: http://www.aidsquilt.org

  A community project that provides a memorial for AIDS victims and brings awareness of the epidemic.

UNAIDS

20, Avenue Appia

CH-1211 Geneva 27

Switzerland

Web site: http://www.unaids.org

  A global organization that is fighting to bring awareness about the AIDS epidemic.

Web Sites

Due to the changing nature of Internet links, Rosen Publishing has developed an online list of Web sites related to the subject of this book. This site is updated regularly. Please use this link to access the list:

http://www.rosenlinks.com/faq/aihi

For Further Reading

Andriote, John-Manuel. *Victory Deferred: How AIDS Changed Gay Life in America.* Chicago: University of Chicago Press, 1999.

Banish, Roslyn. *Focus on Living: Portraits of Americans with HIV and AIDS.* Amherst, MA: University of Massachusetts Press, 2003.

Barnett, Tony, and Alan Whiteside. *AIDS in the Twenty-First Century: Disease and Globalization.* New York, NY: Palgrave Macmillan, 2003.

Bartlett, John G., and Ann K. Finkbeiner. *The Guide to Living with HIV Infection.* Baltimore, MD: John Hopkins University Press, 2006.

Bastos, Christiana. *Global Responses to AIDS: Science in Emergency.* Bloomington, IN: Indiana University Press, 1999.

Gifford, Allen, Kate Lorig, Diana Laurent, and Virginia Gonzalez. *Living Well with HIV & AIDS.* Boulder, CO: Bull Publishing, 2005.

Kalichman, Seth C., ed. *Positive Prevention: Reducing HIV Transmission Among People Living with HIV/AIDS.* New York, NY: Springer Publishing, 2006.

Lather, Patti. *Troubling the Angels: Women Living with HIV/AIDS.* Jackson, TN: Westview Press, 1997.

Schoub, Barry D. *AIDS and HIV in Perspective: A Guide to Understanding the Virus and Its Consequences.* Cambridge, UK: Cambridge University Press, 1999.

Ward, Darrell. *The AmFAR AIDS Handbook: The Complete Guide to Understanding HIV and AIDS.* New York: W. W. Norton, 1999.

Index

A
abstinence, 28
antiretroviral medications, 42, 44
asymptomatic infection, 19
AVERT, 28

B
birth control, choosing, 23
blood transfusions, 11, 13, 21

C
CD4 count, 39–41, 42, 44
condoms, 14, 24, 25, 28–30

D
dental dams, 26, 28, 31
diet and exercise, 46–47
DNA, 16, 17
doctor visits, 39–41, 44
drug resistance tests, 41

F
fidelity, 31
fusion inhibitors, 43
Fuzeon, 43

G
gay-related immunodeficiency
    (GRID), 10

H
hemophiliacs, 10

high-risk behavior, avoiding,
    24, 47–48
HIV/AIDS
  definition of, 6
  genetics of, 15–17
  history of, 9–13
  how it is transmitted, 13,
      14–15, 23, 24, 25
  and life expectancy, 19–20, 22
  myths and facts about, 21–22
  stages of, 18–19
  statistics, 4, 19–20, 26, 28, 32
  symptoms of, 17–18
  testing for, 13, 31–35
  treatment for, 41–44
Hofmann, Regan, 37
home tests, 33–34
homosexual men, 10

I
integrate, 17
intravenous drug users/use, 10,
    15, 21–22, 23, 26, 47, 48

J
Johnson, Magic, 36

K
Kaposi's sarcoma, 9

L
lymph nodes, 18

N

needles, sharing/dirty, 10, 13, 15, 21–22, 24, 26–28, 47, 49
nonnucleoside reverse tran-scriptase inhibitors (NNRTIs), 42, 43
nonoxynol-9, 28–29
nucleoside reverse transcriptase inhibitors (NRTIs), 42–43

O

organ donations, 11

P

Pneumocystis carinii pneumonia (PCP), 9, 19
post-exposure prophylaxis (PEP), 24
protease inhibitors, 43

R

retroviruses, 16
reverse transcriptase, 17, 42
RNA, 16, 17

S

safe sex, 28–31
seroconversion, 19
Stirling, Mark, 4
superinfection, 48
support groups, 38, 49–50, 51
symptomatic infection, 19

U

unprotected sex, 23, 24, 25–26, 47, 49

V

viral load test, 39–41, 42

About the Author
Richard Robinson is a writer of nonfiction books for teens.

Photo Credits
Cover © G.DeGrazia/Custom Medical Stock Photo; p. 5 © Ed Murray/ Star-Ledger/Corbis; p. 7 © George Goodwin/SuperStock; p. 11 © Taro Yamasaki/Time & Life Pictures/Getty Images; p. 12 © Bill Pierce/ Time & Life Pictures/Getty Images; p. 16 © Eye of Science/Photo Researchers, Inc.; p. 20 © Mike Nelson/AFP/Getty Images; pp. 25, 27 © Chip Somodevilla/Getty Images; p. 30 © Seth Perlman/AP Images; p. 32 © Stephen Chernin/Getty Images; p. 34 © Rob Crandall/The Image Works; p. 37 © www.istockphoto.com/Quavondo Nguyen; p. 40 © Tom McCarthy/Photo Network/Alamy; p. 43 © Stephen Shaver/AFP/Getty Images; p. 47 © www.istockphoto.com/Loic Bernard; p. 50 CDC; p. 53 © Norbert Schwerin/The Image Works; pp. 54–55 © David McNew/Getty Images.

Designer: Evelyn Horovicz; Editor: Beth Bryan
Photo Researcher: Amy Feinberg